Holding FORTH

Best Wishes from
[illegible] Ada Bayfield

Ada Bayfield

Published by Ada Bayfield
Henry Bell Close, Gaywood
King's Lynn, Norfolk.

ISBN 0 9522971 0 8

Cover illustration: Scott Wright

Produced by Jim Baldwin
Commercial and Private Publisher,
Fakenham, Norfolk.

Printed in Great Britain.

A Product of Fakenham.

This epistle is dedicated to Deborah Ely who sorted this original muddle out and also to the various voluntary bodies such as the Womens Institute together with all the unsung heroes who worked so hard.

I also hope this will bring pleasure to the now ageing folk who I cared for in my more youthful days, especially the past mothers who struggled through the years to raise their offspring.

The ladies are the backbone of England!

Finally, it is in fond memory of my Downs Syndrome daughter Helen, now sadly departed, but leaving memories for a lot of people who knew her.

Ada Bayfield.

CHILDHOOD MEMORIES

1915, October 18th. I was born in Brixton, I would think rather unexpectedly during a Zeppelin Raid. What my parents were doing in London, apparently for a short stay, I do not know, especially when I was expected – maybe I came early? As it so often happens, there is no stopping a birth.

My sister Athaliah was then thirteen months old and lived with my grandparents at Harpley Mills – the Norman family, my father's parents and brothers and sisters.

My mother Laura was of gipsy origin – the true gipsies in those days. A lot of the big Boswell family are interred at Skegness where most of them lived. There was a large family, very strictly brought up. My mother died when she was 33 years of age. My father died in 1917 also young. His name was Hugh. My sister was named Athaliah Priscilla (Athie for short) after the Maternal Grandmother, what a name. I was named Ada Emily Mary, after Aunts I think from both families.

My father Hugh had been brought up one of seven children as a Methodist. Grandad Norman, William was a local preacher when they lived at Harpley, and was the instigator of the Gospel Hall built on a piece of land given by the late Lord Cholmondeley of Houghton Hall, who helped to fund it. My father was going into the Ministry after the 1914–1918 war was over – he was not called up as he helped his father at the mill. He was also I imagine somewhat delicate as I think during 1917 after a 'flu epidemic he contracted pneumonia and eventually tuberculosis, from which he did not recover. Not surprising as there were no antibiotics or special treatment in those days, I should think a lot of them died from exposure as they spent their days in a hut outside.

My mother was, I think, an Evangelist and travelled around for the Temperance people who I call 'Down with the drink folk'. Eventually called the 'White Ribbon', as far as I know it is still going strongly to convert the drinkers.

She met Hugh my father on visiting Harpley and they must have married pretty quickly as they were in their late twenties. Hugh died at Burnham Overy and is interred there. My mother took us to live at Gosforth near Newcastle, one of her brothers lived there. He was a painter and decorator I believe. I can remember the house we lived in, as my mother was away a great deal we had a housekeeper to look after us. Nobody stayed very long as I was a really naughty and problem child. One housekeeper I can remember, the last one, wore a long purple dress which rustled – I suppose it was taffeta.

Occasionally our Aunt Linda, my mother's sister, came to look after us – very houseproud and smart. When at four years of age I can remember her teaching us to wash up properly, no running water in those days. After the pots and pans had been washed with some sort of soda or soap we had to rinse them.

I can remember my mother taking us to have our photographs taken in Newcastle – I had used the scissors not very aptly and chopped a bit out of my fringe. We also used to go to Jesmond Dene occasionally – like a park then, I remember it was very green and flowery.

Eventually we went to Boarding School in Berwick-on-Tweed, St. Rolands. I can remember eating a lot of tripe and porridge (I have never eaten tripe since). My sister was very unwell and did not eat much. I have always had a stomach like a horse – so thrived quite well (a good grounding for my future nursing career). I do not remember how long we were there as time means nothing to the young ones!!

I can remember going for crocodile walks every day over the grass dunes down by the sea. We used to bathe in a pool with a stone wall around it. The water always seemed to be cold, it is a wonder my sister survived!

We wore navy dresses with white collars and navy reefer coats and hats with red badges. On Sundays we wore cream serge coats and navy fluffy hats – beaver I think, white socks and black patent shoes – Ugh! How I hated it all. I was a dirty child, I have never been very partial to posh clothes and still dress for comfort.

My mother realized she had not much longer to live and went to see a specialist, so had to make arrangements for Athie and myself to be cared for. It was her wish and in her will that we should be cared for in Norfolk by my father's people – the Normans.

By this time Grandad, who had retired from Harpley Mills, bought a house in King's Lynn in Avenue Road. My Grandmother wasn't in the best of health, but two Aunts lived with them. Aunt Annie was a trained nurse and did her Midwifery at Queen Charlotte's Hospital in London and practised privately with the consultant doing general and midwifery – a private nurse who stayed in patients' houses, living in when the occasion warranted. Aunt Grace the youngest daughter, a lovely gentle soul with a great sense of humour, kept house.

The last time we saw our mother was at Peterborough Station where Aunt Annie, who was made our guardian, met us and our enormous cabin trunk with our belongings. We were too young to know what was happening to us – and of course had a good few upheavals in our short lives. I have thought since becoming a mother myself what she must have felt like, she must have been a very brave woman with great faith.

Well, as my sister was so delicate, and more room for us, we went to live with the eldest daughter Emily, who had been tragically widowed just before we arrived. Wereham was a lovely village, it still is except for some changes. I can remember it as the happiest days of my life.

I was seven years old and my sister eight years. Aunt Emmie's son Norman ran the family farm, her other son Teddy died when they had a bakers business at Massingham, he was only seventeen. Her only daughter, whom we call cousin Emmie, also lived some of the time with us. She was a very clever lady in accountancy and until we lost her at the age of 86 was an energetic and accomplished person.

Farming in those days after the 1914 war was not very profitable, my Aunt must have worked very hard to make ends meet. She certainly did not benefit from my sister and myself as I believe it was ten shillings per week for both of us.

We had a wonderful childhood and even working hard doing our chores benefited from good plain food. My sister gradually began to eat more and had Scotts Emulsion to 'vitimanise' her. I believe I had cod liver oil and malt every Friday night. I usually had to have it as I ate all sorts of things, like half grown apples. We had an orchard with a big wall all around and a locked door, but, as I was a wonderful climber was able to climb over the calves shed roof and shin down the tree – oh the joy of it – but even the terrible bowel deterrent liquorice powder, didn't stop me. Whoever invented that stuff should have been shot. Syrup of figs was nice to take but after effects perhaps not so pleasant.

The lovely days of summer – hard winters, we could walk miles when fine, at least I did, Athie was not quite up to it. When you think how free we were to enjoy the simple pleasures of the country side with no real dangers for us. No wonder I hated school, it did cramp your style a bit. Luckily we both had learned to read and write while away at boarding school as most children did not start school in the old days until they were 4½ or 5 years old. A child in a normal happy household will learn enough without being pushed into playschools, unless there is some difficulty in their make-up. These modern days there are more deficiency problems than in our young days, so they do perhaps need that help.

Family life is so important and parents who do not want to look after their offspring should not have them – it is selfish.

By contrast to today it was a tough life in our early days, but we were happy and never really missed our parents. Children if brought up within the rules and affection of their family take it all in their stride and never panic in an emergency – they have a good start which does help them when they get older. Farming was hard in those days with very little profit, but everything has compensations.

Athie and myself before going to school arose early, did our ablutions in cold water, jug and ewer on the wash stand, often icy in the winter (a good excuse for me not to wash)!

After a breakfast of good bread and dripping or marmalade and jam, and of course lovely dairy butter (I never eat margarine even now if I can help it), we made our beds then I took three cans of fresh lovely milk to three places down the road, Flegg Green, including Mr. and Mrs. Wells the school master and mistress in the bungalow. I was terrified of her (the only one I might add) but like him I now know why he had a twinkle in his eye when he spoke to me! I loved to walk in the dykes instead of the road.

My sister slept in a double bed but I had to have a single one as I was so naughty. The windows faced the back and the scullery roof led down, to help me with my climbing out when I was sent to bed for my wickedness. But I had plenty of reading books under the mattress so I never really suffered.

We were 10 minutes' walk away from school, which had two large classrooms and a small backroom for infants, who were taught by a pupil teacher, God help her. The girls were taught by Mrs. Wells and the boys by Mr. Wells, but tuition was good. The only means of heating was a coke monk stove and for the middle of the morning the children who were considered delicate had hot milk, which was kept hot on top of the stove – Athie didn't like it as it was very creamy! I hated school and discipline but did like English and Art, so did quite well I think.

But eventually I was sent to King's Lynn to live with my Grandparents and was made to make the effort to get a bit of 'learning' in to me as we say in Norfolk.

What I really enjoyed after helping with the housework etc., and especially in the holidays was helping on the farm and roaming in the fields (no fear in those days) there wasn't a tree I could not climb – especially if I needed to escape punishment!

I can only once remember having a stick across my bottom and it was Easter time. We all went in the pony and trap to the Easter Celebration called the Service of Song held at Boughton Village Chapel, about four miles away, and afterwards had tea at the farmhouse with the people who were the upstanding support of the Chapel. I always had a feeling of not being welcome and would wander off after tea, of course I realized now why. I was no doubt frowned upon as the Imp of Satan, but they were nice kind people. Anyway Athie and myself loved the ride. No cars in those days, only the village doctor who had a funny little two seater and a dickie at the back. He must have worked very hard and looking back can remember my Aunt and cousin deciding he was not always in control of himself – but I am sure he needed a little drop of sustenance to enable him to survive. Dr. Steele was a great believer in purging the inner man and I am sure it saved a lot of time for the hospitals. After eating too many green apples he made me very ill with his treatment!

To go back to the Easter episode, when we went to the Easter Service of Song, we wore our best clothes. Athie always got ready first and myself last, as I seemed to hate being dressed up, and still do! Somehow I went down to our walled-in fruit and vegetable garden, climbing over the calves shed roof and down the nearest tree, we had cream serge coats, black beaver hats and still cream socks and black patent shoes, which was our Sunday outfit at Boarding School. I know after I had my fill I heard my cousin Norman shouting for me, looked at my coat all green and took off as if the Devil was behind me, chased by Norman with a stick.

Now it must have been providence because I was saved by our gander (we were birds of a feather), we had the care of him and his wives while the dear old farmer Billy had to go into hospital with a strangulated hernia – he was a character, and have thought since what great entertainment he must have been.

The gander had taken a dislike to Norman so very wrathfully he chased him away. So much for burglar alarms when geese are around!! I had to go to the outing in my soiled coat but clean socks.

Regarding Billy and Martha Mee – she sang in the Church Choir, they never altered the clock, which had just started to change then, but after being late for church once managed to get thereafter at the right time.

I still maintain and it is the only old fashioned thought, that barring the facts of life, it is much better if you live in the country, especially on a farm. We all had to work quite hard, I loved it much better than housework and school.

We had lovely long summers, usually May to end of September I think, and during the summer holidays helped with the Harvest. We had a horse called *Bouncer*, he was huge and strong and used to pull the wagon at Haytime and Harvest, he was lovely. I used to ride on him, mind you when he used to stop on our way home and wanted a drink, which he had in our pond, I often slipped over his head, but never drowned. He never went too far in – the reason I think.

I used to take the cows down to the field about two miles away which we owned called the Wash Pits and fetched them home in the afternoon for milking – only in the summer. We had a black Heifer called *Polly* – they all had names and she was expecting her first calf. I knew our cows, but I found out why our prize bull used to serve the cows. An old farmer, horrible old man, used to bring his cows to be served, our cows were always brushed and groomed before milking and well fed but his were skinny – he had the usual red face due to over indulging. One day when he came I was up the yard and the pen where the 'marital performance' took place was handy and I happened to be up one of the fruit trees and saw the procedure. Now children are very sensible and do not panic (unlike adults) and I was very interested, and can remember, when our *Polly* has her calf, where will it come out? It is a big animal, even if a calf. However, when *Polly* was getting nearer her time, she was getting very plump and a bit slow walking, I took her down to the Wash Pits in the morning after milking, Norman said if she was all right to leave her there for the night. When I got there to fetch the cows up *Polly* was not all right, and not going in to any details was silently 'heaving' so I brought her home with the cows. Yes, I was a bit worried, although by this time put two and two together and had an idea from which part of her body it would appear.

I was on the horse and after a few stops and starts got her to the end of the first lane, now there was to be a quick think on intuition you might say. I must get help quickly. At the bottom of the lane lived a family, father was the village cobbler, he had a wooden leg (they were wooden in those days) strapped on. He rode a bicycle, I don't know how. I told him not to stop to put his leg on but to come and the answer was very quickly 'how the hell am I going to ride me bike without two legs' I never forgot it. He sent me home to tell Norman to get ready and he would bring the cows home. I will never forget that ride, for about ¼ mile it would be. I galloped along (I would have made a good jockey) my Aunt was near the kitchen window and saw me. I kept going and shouted 'Mr. Carter is bringing the cows home and *Polly*'. She hollered (she could holler well my Aunt) 'put the horse up and get back here'. I had no intention of 'getting back here'. This was the most exciting thing of the day, I think I was 10 years old or nearly. I think in the rush I was forgotten, I believe we had the vet – but I saw my first insight into midwifery. Now I think everything to get a baby, pregnancy and labour is awful but . . . to see a new life come in to the world is wonderful, it has lived with me all my life, even after delivering a few thousand babies, wanted and unwanted. It has always given me a wondrous feeling even after a few hair-raising experiences. It is still with me and I fully understand that birth and death are inevitable.

OUR FOLK The day the District Nurse was removed from her house and the care of her villagers, was the worst occurrence that ever happened. She was the adviser, healer, counsellor and a friend to all, and, as needed, very strict and persuasive in her advice.

Our house was a centre for her at times, also a house in Front Street, Wereham, had a room for the doctor who came from Fincham, as well as Dr. Steele from Stoke Ferry.

Compulsory vaccination for smallpox had started, unless a form was signed by your G.P. to the contrary. We had an outbreak of Encephalitis Lethargica, namely 'sleepy sickness', a virus in some cases fatal, but a vaccine was found. Unless really acute, such as appendicitis etc., very few were admitted to hospital. There was a Nursing Association until after the 1939–1945 war where people who could pay did so according to their circumstances. Children I believe were exempt, and the Orphans Pension was 10 shillings per week from the state.

There was a lot of poverty as there always seems to be, but everybody helped out. Abuse of children always seemed to be nipped in the bud. More later on. There was a little bit of scandal now and then but it does help to keep the world turning.

RELIGION The Chapel was situated by the pond in the village near the Post Office and school, there was a separate Sunday School next to the Chapel, I often wondered why. My family being Methodist attended 'religiously' Sunday School in the morning and Chapel in the afternoon and evening. Due to unavoidable circumstance, Nursing and what have you, I was never able to keep this pace up, but what a grounding!

After morning Sunday School, Athie and myself and two sisters from the Post Office and sometimes from the bakers (churchgoers I might add) were allowed to go for a walk round the Row if weather permitted, it must have been three miles, but we usually got home for dinner. I never had dry feet as I preferred to walk in the dykes, much softer than the rough roads.

After Chapel in the afternoon, the local Preacher used to come to ours for high tea. All on best behaviour and the Sunday pink china used. I hated Sundays. But what wonderful people the local preachers were – people used to come from other villages on their bicycles, sidecars, motor bikes or walked unless they had a pony and trap like we had.

Our organ was a pump affair and poor old Bob Rogers used to pump it but in the very hot weather would nod off to sleep. My Aunt and cousin who played used to have to poke him to arouse him. Actually we had one preacher, Billy Pearman, who loudly sang and acclaimed the Lord and brought Hell Fire into his sermons – he scared me to death as I really thought I would be given to the Devil for being such a sinner. So if the music faded, well everybody was happy to let Billy carry on. There was a brother and sister who sat near the front, they were very tall, I never knew how old they were – Martha was an epileptic apparently. I remember her as tightly laced and she wore a little straw hat, she looked very straight up and down. I can remember her one very hot Sunday having one of her seizures! I nudged my sister Athie as by now there was a funny noise – she is going to have a fit, most exciting, no panic. She was conveyed to the porch by two males with my Aunt and another female leading the procession. The loud singing of Billy's favourite hymn (and mine) *All Hail the Power of Jesu's Name*, just went on. Now as I have learned she would be out for the count. Sleeping, then while help was sought to take her home, the said ladies undid her tight collar and the most fascinating thing for me was her corsets! Whalebone I should say and behold the dear soul was quite plump around the middle, bless her, I was never afraid of fits in humans during my whole life. We had our frailer brethren, a few retarded in some way. But they grew up with us and were accepted.

Sunday School Anniversary was the only service I enjoyed once a year in the summer. Best straw hats trimmed with flowers (tolerated needless to say) and best Sunday frocks. Plenty of singing and recitations – lovely days.

Long summer days and holiday for Harvest, everybody worked hard – adults and children. I loved riding on the horse *Bouncer*. My Aunt used to send food by Athie for us all. The favourite cake was Harvest Field cake, like rock cake but softer and larger and richer, filled with fruit and good dairy butter. I still eat butter and only ate margarine when we were rationed during the 1939 war years whilst nursing.

My favourite pastime when taking the cows to the pasture would be collecting caterpillars which I kept in boxes with leaves, anyway they seemed to live and become chrysalises which I put in matchboxes and hid in various nooks in the large dining-room which was used on Holy days, I has a wonderful collection of moths and butterflies which I let go eventually in case they were confiscated.

Toadstools – I once put some in a Christmas cracker box in the big box room upstairs, and after a dreadful smell they were discovered by my Aunt who turned them out.

My Aunt used to have a separator in our dairy where the cream was separated from the milk. Once a week the cream was made into butter by a large churn and then with the wooden pats made into 1 lb and ½ lbs of lovely butter. My aunt once won a prize for her butter made in the shape of the Prince of Wales Feathers coat of arms. I should say this was at the Royal Norfolk show. The Royal Norfolk show was held every five years but the annual show was in the Walks, it cost five shillings to go in.

The only bus I can remember was from Methwold, Carters I think, and we had our Sunday School outing to the seaside every summer to Hunstanton. I can remember us getting stuck half way up the hill and we all pushed it and got it going. We took lots of food and fluid including non-alcoholic ginger beer, which was made at home. Masons were the producers and tea and buns were given to us at Hunstanton Methodist Sunday School – Oh what lovely days, it is a pity we have to grow up, I suppose I did learn a bit at school, but to my horror was suddenly uprooted and sent to live with my grandparents and two aunts, one of whom was our guardian Annie, the trained nurse – I still have one of her case books.

Well I did learn a lot – not so much at school except basic items and discipline, but managed to learn a few more facts of life from Avenue Road where we lived. Whilst residing at Lynn the house seemed to become a hospital – a lot of operations were performed at home if suitable on the kitchen table, dressings sterilized in the oven, I think, and all the instruments boiled. Mr. Plowright the doctor was a clever surgeon and I remember my Grandfather, who had a long white beard, which my Aunt used to plait. When he was ill he had his bladder operation in the usual two stages, he did well – no antibiotics or transfusions in those days. The open ether and chloroform was the unpleasant part! I don't think anyone died on the kitchen table and Grandad was up and about in a month; he was nearly eighty years old. My sister had her tonsils out there the same year, and as she seemed to get a lot of fussing and gifts I wished I could have mine out. I had to wait until I was 13 and had it done in hospital, the cheek of it, maybe it was safer.

My Grandmother always wore black and seemed to be an invalid, she travelled around in a bath chair with a steering handle. She had had a largish family, but died at 79, I think just before Grandad. I used to ride in the bath-chair sometimes when we used to go to chapel – in Tower Street in those days. Grandad used to wear a little skull cap on his head as he said he felt the draught blowing on his bald pate!

Well, all good things come to an end, my sister became a nurse-maid, she must have felt very homesick to go away, although one of my mother's sisters looked after her as she had her first job with a nice Italian family.

I had learnt shorthand and typewriting, that was a waste of time and money, but my Aunt Annie thought I might be suitable for nursing. If ever I join her upstairs I will ask her where she got the idea! You did not start until you were 18 years of age, time enough I should say. You were taken to be interviewed by the Matron when you were 17 years old I think, and she liked us all to do other jobs in the meantime. (I should say in case you changed your mind.) I did the Christmas serving at W. H. Smith's, which I enjoyed and then really got into the profession at the deep end!

INTRODUCTION TO NURSING

We had a Nursing Home on London Road which catered for private patients, including emergency midwifery now and then. I was hired as a dogsbody to wait on the secretary, she was wonderful, I was a bit in awe of her. We had our own x-ray and a consultant who took the place of Dr. Plowright. He was a Mr. C. E. S. Jackson, a big man and very clever and hard working. I was frightened to death of him, but survived. We had a nice theatre and anterooms, the Matron used to run it with the help of trained staff who had completed their training at the General Hospital and needed to earn money and experience. As far as I know there is only one still with us, older than me but a great character.

Mr. Jackson had a chauffeur, just as well as he seemed to be working 24 hours a day. When he went out operating in the houses he took one of the staff, complete with equipment, which I put in the car. I think it was a Rolls or a Bentley, occasionally I had to go with them to make sure all was complete.

I had to clean the instruments when we brought them back and strip the dressing drums. I learnt a lot then and enjoyed the variety, I do not think I was much of an asset to the secretary. Well, the time came near to start my training. Incidentally when my Aunt took me for my interview with the Matron, I can see her now not very tall, and as I found out very religious. But remember her as having large false teeth. I was issued with material for uniform enough for 14 aprons, 7 dresses, 4 caps and collars and cuffs. The grey and white striped dresses were lovely material and until a few years ago had a scrubbing apron which I cherished. The same colour and stripes as the dresses. I of course due to old bones am unable to kneel now. I was not sure if I would be able to tolerate all the rules and regulations.

Although she was strict she was a wonderful clever Matron, very just and kind. We need them now. No 'hanky panky' as my Grandad would say. It seemed with that Female Asset the hospital proceeded like clockwork, and really when you are still young whatever goes on in the world it does not bother you. Ignorance is bliss sometimes.

King's Lynn General Hospital became an official Training School the year when about 12 of us started. The Norfolk and Norwich being already such. No Preliminary Training School, P.T.S., but we had to present ourselves to the Home Sister cum House Keeping Sister, and Catering and Deputy to Matron, i.e. Assistant Matron, small but very plump like a cottage loaf, and very kind. She thoroughly inspected us, rigged out in our uniform dresses, well below the knee, I believe the reason being on bending forward we must not expose too much leg. Our hair well tucked up under our caps, as it should be now. After all patients under our care do not want hair flapping over them, let alone the danger of the nurses picking up the 'dickies' from a patient! Black shoes and stockings, but I did not mind them really. Then we were escorted to the wards and presented to the Sister in charge where we were to labour. Myself not quite 18 for a few weeks, I was deposited on the Children's Ward so would not be contaminated by the male community. Actually we had a semi private ward attached, three two-bedded ones. Four had to attend a mixed consignment of bodies!

The Sister was Welsh, Miss Jones, very excitable and energetic, her first words to me were, 'I will endeavour to train you to be like your dear Aunt!' I should have run away then and there!

Each Ward had a Sister, a fourth year nurse who acted as Staff Nurse or when trained stayed on for a time. There were no Orderlies or Auxiliaries, except in the Army. So there were 1st, 2nd, 3rd and 4th year nurses and one maid for each ward. The Men's and Women's Wards, long ones, but there seemed to be plenty of room between them and the lockers. We used screens, extra work but much cleaner than curtains. There were two wards on the Men's Wards and three on the Women's Wards and a small Special Ward for Midwifery.

All our babies were born at home, except for anything very abnormal, until the 1930s. Queen Charlottes of course was just a midwifery one in London.

We had a nice Nurses Home. Should be so nowadays and much safer and cheaper. We were called to go on duty in the morning at about 6 a.m. by the Night Sister, who rang a large bell, like a ship's bell. We had to strip our beds, not make them and report in the Hospital dining-room. Our names were ticked off by Night Sister in a large book, much better than clocking in. If anyone was missing, not very often mind you, the dining-room maid was sent off to the Home Sister to enquire the reason for absence. Night Sister served porridge and hot breakfast of some sort and tea. Then at 6.50 a.m. Matron came in to pray (she came without her teeth once) and I truly believe she prayed we would stay the 10–12 hour working day. We had an hour, eventually 1½ hours, off duty when we attended our lectures. We had a day off each week, but had to attend the Consultant lectures.

Mr. Jackson was General and Urinary and Obstetrician, eventually Mr. Lewin, Ear Nose and Throat and general surgery. One Resident Registrar, Miss White, very clever, eventually went to the Royal Free Hospital. Miss Elsie Johnson did the Medical side and relieved Miss White when necessary. She became a General Practitioner at Downham Market. How they all worked, day and night, and found time to enjoy life. The few local General Practitioners used to come in to entertain each other. There was a Dr. Lisle Punch who had a practice in Wimpole Street, London and his Hospital Appointments. He was a very clever man and gave us our Consultant Medicine Lectures. I believe he was shell shocked during the 1914–1918 War, as he appeared to be very fidgety, sniffed a lot and danced about a bit. He was eventually replaced by Dr. Holmes Walkins, he as well as being a chest man, especially Tuberculosis, took over the Medicine Lectures.

During the morning up to 9.30–10 a.m. 1st year nurses did the cleaning of the lockers and helped with washing the patients and bed making, false teeth seemed to be cleaned by us and put in the patients' tooth mugs. We had a few Irish girls doing their training and one of them was like myself, a bit 'scatty' and somehow got the teeth mixed up, I cannot remember what happened, but imagine the chaos. We went to the dining-room during the morning for 20 minutes and had bread and dripping and it was good. I think the Nurses Home Maids made the beds because of our inspection by Home Sister.

First Year Nurses had a good grounding, cleaning on the wards, trollies, sluices, bathrooms and toilets, the Ward Maid did the floors, polished with a 'dumpty', scrubbed I believe once weekly. Our last meal was at 8.30 p.m. before we went off duty, to be in bed by 10.30 p.m. Home Sister used to come and knock on our door to make sure we were bedded and lights out. But what went on after that when we had our little meetings in our rooms, I think she turned a deaf ear to.

We had plain but good food and the same with the patients, Miss Gleave the Assistant Matron sorted the diets out in the big kitchen. We had a female cook, I always think females wash their hands more frequently than chefs, and quite honestly we never seemed to have infections.

We had a Septic Ward (St. Nicholas) downstairs, people with septic limbs and a lot of horrible complaints were admitted there. We had a small theatre there so they never went near our large lovely theatre upstairs.

We had one Night Sister on duty at night, I do not know how on earth she managed, she eventually had a Staff Nurse with her. She managed Casualty at night with the help of a junior nurse who was a runner. There were two on night duty to run between the wards, as each ward had a 2nd and 3rd year nurse in charge. The runner had to help with the 'backs' patients pressure points and general nursing. She relieved the nurse for half an hour in the night for a meal, which was eaten in the ward kitchen. I remember going down to the big kitchen, very large and recently extended and equipped, just before I started. It even had a large hot plate oven where the stew (good stuff) and vegetables were kept hot and a sweet, I believe good rice pudding, sometimes steamed puddings and custard and all carried on a large wooden tray, phew!! I well remember coming down the corridor to St. Nicholas Ward one summer and the doors were open near the river and a rat ran over my foot. I dropped the tray and you can imagine the mess. Night Sister heard, she had double hearing. She came of course and gave me a good talking to. With her very large bunch of keys (after I had cleared up) took me to the inner sanctum of the kitchen and cupboards, I had to cook bacon and eggs for dinner and I think took cake round as well. Oh what joy!

How Matron managed with 50 plus nurses in training to cover the wards I do not know. There was a board in her office with all our names on. She knew exactly where we should be labouring. Changed over every three months on each department, including O.P.D, etc. Only the three months on night duty at one time it worked out.

We eventually had a tutor, but Mrs. Gleave gave us our Nursing and Hygiene lectures, Matron gave our Anatomy and Physiology and the Consultants Medical and Surgical. After two years this included six weeks as junior in the theatre, that was a nightmare. We had our first State Preliminary Examination which we had to pass before going on to 'higher things'. Before we sat our first State, Matron used to invite us up to her flat after duty for extra tuition. We were not forced to go but very few were absent. We either went to the Norfolk and Norwich or London for firstly a written exam and a fortnight later oral and practical. I do not need to tell you how we felt, but we made up for it and had a meal out (not so expensive in those days) and enjoyed ourselves before coming back by train.

On Sunday evenings Matron and Miss Gleave held a service in the Nurses Home sitting-room after duty; we sang hymns from the Sankey and Moodie Hymn Book, very rousing it was too. There was one named *Where is my wandering boy tonight* and we requested it for Miss Gleave who we think did not attract the males. I do not know what sort of talk Matron gave as usually we fell asleep.

My second insight into midwifery came in my 2nd year, of course Abnormal Midwifery. Our Special Ward for Eclamptic, very ill high blood pressure mothers in the late stages of Toxaemia, fitting. One lady who had had her family, four or five, at home was admitted. She had had with her other pregnancies quite good Antenatal treatment by the District Nurse and Doctor, but I think this one was an afterthought (no birth control in those days, a ticket to Hunstanton and got off at Heacham) and was afraid to notify anyone of her plight. However, she appeared to have more than one infant in her inner sanctum. We did not have many multiple pregnancies, except twins, so Mr. Jackson, our Consultant was called in, as I have said a great man also in stature and took one look and said (he boomed) we will wait and see what will come forth. I will not go into details about sedation and treating the mother, but with help from his Lordship she came into labour and eventually there were three puny little ones, alive miraculously. We had no incubators in those days, but Shock Cradles with electric bulbs to keep the babies warm. They were wrapped in gauze, too expensive to produce now, but wonderful, their bodies quickly oiled and yes, we had oxygen to give them, but the best method of resuscitation as a last resort was a few drops of brandy on the tongue after the air passage was cleared (it was good brandy in those days and kept in the medicine cupboard under lock and key for lighting the Christmas puddings), and of course a good old gasp from the baby and with luck if the brain was functioning, breathing established slowly, and let me tell you NO ill effects, as no fiddling about. The mother did recover and as far as I knew the babies also. There were no antibiotics still but by 1936/7 M & B 693 tablets and Prentizol, the first trial of penicillin, bright pink in colour became available and had to be given by syringe in large dosages.

Of course there were after effects, but with these (badly infected limbs, some amputated, septic abortions, etc), it was a matter of life and death and as far as I can remember it worked in most cases, eventually of course Dr. Fleming and others medicated it with easier results.

Our x-ray was donated by Lord Fermoy of Sandringham, we were still a Voluntary Hospital until the end of the 1945 War. Blood was only infused where it was needed desperately and you had to have a donor to match up. The Path. Lab. dealt with that and the Hospital Doctors. Our drip apparatus was a Heath Robinson affair but worked very well. I cannot remember anyone being killed off with Transfusion. How easy it is now to have Drip Sets ready. We had a lovely Theatre with Anaesthetists Room, sterilized room for setting trolleys. I still believe in boiling as much as possible. And a Scrubbing room where the dressings were and where doctors scrubbed and were gowned. Mr. Jackson had to have a large gown and cap, gloves and white rubber boots, I used to tremble when I tied him up, bless him. He was the best surgeon ever, even if irritable at times, but never shall we see his like again, especially for fast surgery, big operations as well, and of course had to control bleeding which could not be replaced. Mr. Lewin eventually arrived, which greatly helped and then Mr. J. O. Harrison, quite young, as Mr. Jackson retired. Both were excellent, only two to cover that hospital, 250–300 beds. The Anaesthetists were trainee local Doctors in practice who shared the job. I cannot describe the senior lady who used to come but she was a character.

The Children's Ward was the saddest one. Very badly burned and scalded children, not child abuse. One little boy who I think lives near Spalding had terrible burns, Dickie Hammond, and he was in for a long time, but recovered. I often wondered how he fared, he was my pet and I was the one to do things for him.

I was developing an infected appendix while nearly ready to take my State Finals, but just managed to make the two journeys and visits, luckily it was Norwich again.

I by this time was back in Theatre struggling to learn how to assist at operations as the Senior Staff Nurse was leaving. Getting up at night in turn with Theatre Sister, she was wonderful but very disliked as bad tempered, had thyroid trouble. I was in awe of her. We passed our finals except for three or four and were asked to stay on as Staff Nurses. Usually for about a year because you booked up for your midwifery a year before. My Aunt wanted me to go to Queen Charlottes where she trained. I did not want to and towards the end of my year, I was stuck in theatre and developed thyroid trouble, family complaint and had six weeks off for rest and operation, enough said. Having to have a Local Anaesthetic to start and even with sedation, flat on the theatre table with a sandbag under my neck, I thought I would never come out alive, and was being paid back by the Holy Man above for all my past wicked ways. However, eventually anaesthetized and after a few ups and downs recovered.

Told by Dr. Walkins the Medical Man and Mr. Lewin advised me not to do my Midwifery, but by now there were two modern hospitals opened up in and out of London. So booked in at the Perivale Maternity Hospital, Greenford on the Western Avenue. So had some months to fill in, advised to take an easy job, I ask you? But a friend who trained with me was working at the Evelyn Nursing Home at Cambridge to earn a bit more money. We only got £60.00. per year for being a Staff Nurse in Hospital, it went a hell of a long way.

She suggested I might apply the nursing home in Cambridge in Brooklands Avenue, which was to close down in a few months.

PASTURES NEW

So off I went, just had to send a reference and no interview as such, very trusting I might say. I arrived there on the said day, met the Matron who owned it, actually I found she was not trained, but a very nice elderly soul who received me with open arms. She took me to my room and handed me the keys for my wardrobe, where I was to keep all the drugs. Oh yes, nobody pinched drugs in those days, at least I wasn't aware of it and did not really bother as I had the keys. I was there for about four months, mostly medical nursing and small operations in our small theatre as such. But social life, that lady made sure I had my share of outside interests, I think she tried to match me up. Luckily for the first time in my life, as I had just returned from a visit with one of my colleagues whom I had trained with, were invited for three weeks holiday in Bournemouth to stay with one of the two remaining Aunts, sister to my mother.

She had a fabulous house and a nice husband, she married late in life, they were very rich but Dick loved his little drop, but we loved him. His people were the main confectioners in Bournemouth, Parsons the name. He looked after the mill at Christchurch, he used to take us in his Studebaker car there, we used to have a fabulous picnic. He had a friend who had his own private plane, Uncle Dick wouldn't fly, but we had a trip over the fields, sea and the Isle of Wight, this was the 1938 crisis year.

My Aunt rigged me out with a completely new wardrobe and some for my friend and we had few clothes so we felt like princesses. We travelled home among sailors and other call-ups back to London and then to King's Lynn. After a few days, off to Cambridge again, I left Cambridge with some regrets and after a check up on my health at home, took off to Perivale to start my Midwifery, one of the first groups for First and Second part Training, six and nine months at different hospitals.

My Aunt by this time had her own Maternity Home, Holly Lodge in King's Lynn, as the Grandparents had passed on. When I arrived at Liverpool Street Station with overnight case, trunk case having been sent in advance, complete with uniform which we provided, plenty of it as we kept it from our training days, but with a few additions. I got on the underground without a clue really how I was going to get there, but met up with Nurse Harvey from Yarmouth, so had company, we got out at Park Royal Station and went the rest of the way by bus.

What a lovely modern hospital, it hasn't closed that many years ago. Fifty beds, lovely labour wards and theatre, a lovely Scots Matron who received all 12 of us from different parts of the country. We still worked long hours, but had good off duty and well fed. On night duty for the first time, went off sometimes for 1½ hours break to the dining-room, we had a night cook and had a good meal. You were able to play table-tennis or have a rest.

We used to have our Consultants Lectures at Willesden Maternity Hospital, we had to go by taxi. Mr. Arnold Walker was our lecturer, he became Head of the Royal College of Gynaecology and Obstetrics and Chairman of the Central Midwives Board. He did not die very long ago. At his first lecture he said 'To you ladies who wish to become Midwives, just understand that a baby will be born without help and there is no stopping it. I am here to teach you to observe and distinguish the normal from the abnormal, and how to conduct normal labour and be of help to the mother. Every pregnancy, labour and delivery are different, so be on your toes and good luck to you all.' We needed it in the future, the first Consultant Mr. Alan Moncrief, was the first Consultant Paediatrician, became Professor Moncrief, a nice man and like Arnold Walker very humorous. I met up with both in later years.

We used to go to clinics in Ealing Broadway, and went on a train called the Push and Pull. If it was our day off we went to the cinema there. It was Shirley Temple then.

There was the best method of labelling the babies, they were bone necklaces in solution and the letters for naming on, on the admission of the mother and as soon as the baby was born it was put on and sealed and never removed until discharge. They never had sore necks and unlike the terrible plastic bands never came off.

As a lot of new factories had grown up a lot of East End people moved out here, a lot had disproportion of the hips due to rickets in childhood, so plenty of abnormal midwifery. We had to see so many normal deliveries, and then deliver so many under supervision and then in our case books very similar to my late Aunts' book which she like us had to present for our State Exam. Well all good things come to an end and we finished and very sorry to leave with invitation to come back when trained.

Home again for a break staying with my Aunt and cousin, who had left Wereham and lived in Sidney Street, not far from the nursing home. So I helped at the nursing home, but only for a couple of weeks as War was declared in September 1939, I was sent for a bit early for my Second part Midwifery to Walthamstow, Thorpe Coombe Hospital, also fairly modern.

The Government in their so called short sightedness, being men, called up every available nurse, including midwives, who were on the reserve for the forces. We were caught napping as usual, it is a pity Mr. Churchill wasn't P.M. then. Nobody listened to him, but of course, luckily the Labour Government was ousted and he took over with a mixed Government.

I should have gone to the Middlesex for six weeks, but took off in a hurry to Walthamstow, to my horror I was the only Part 2 Pupil Midwife! Thus began 'bedlam'. It was I believe a 50 bedded plus unit, double storey. The top floor was closed during the War. The intake of patients varied as evacuees came hither and thither from the country.

We did nine months training between the Unit and District. I arrived at 5.30 p.m. and was met by the Matron, a nice soul, her arm in a sling. Apparently she had clambered up the sandbags that decorated our bottom windows to save the glass splintering in the windows.

I was taken to the Nurses Home, with was perched at the front on top of a hilly road. She was pleased to see me; I don't wonder when I saw the set up of staff. She asked me if I would mind coming on duty (really to see the set up) so of course I naturally said yes. You never said no while nursing. But as I got wiser in later years, should have said no to many things that are not mentioned. A long corridor met my eyes, longer than that of Perivale, but at least not so many as there are in today's hospitals. Abomination I call it, bad for legs and feet especially, maybe good exercise, which could be put to better purposes. The Labour Wards, I think two, but one had to be adapted as a theatre, which did not matter, but usually two being delivered in each Labour Ward at a time very often. The Labour Ward Sister was on reserve for the Q.E. and eventually was called up for the war activities. Myself being Part 2 became a full grown

Midwife before I should have done. Mind you, when you did get flung out you did feel able to cope with all sorts of conditions. God help us.

We had three months in the Unit, clinics and everything, what a nightmare. I often wonder if the mothers got their right babies. All fed three hourly if under 7 lbs, plastic name tapes, we had a big nursery, so kept the three hourly ones to one side. No room for cots then in the wards and in any case 60% of the mothers were exhausted.

The one Sister on the ward was little and small stature, but had a remarkable temper, mind you she was rather overworked. Like myself needed to be in two places at once. The Registrar was also a remarkable lady and very short tempered, but not to be wondered at. The Junior Doctor was a much quieter lady and very much in awe of her Senior, that made two of us! The Consultant who visited us in emergency came from Middlesex Unit and was Dame Louise Mackliroy. I will not dwell upon my experience with her as too much to tell of other things. I was not in London for the worst of the bombing, but the siren went and in bed all would rise but soon got fed up as losing a lot of sleep anyway, Ah me, what a thing it is to be young, burdens fall lightly on young shoulders (didn't of course know any better).

Life flew on and I had to go to York Road Lying Hospital for my Health and running of the General Social Hygiene and Administrative Tuition and a lot about drainage, etc. I and most of us were so tired when we arrived there, it was our day off, once a fortnight and having lost sleep, etc. were glad to sit down and have a good sleep. I can remember coming back in a Smog, which was London Fog, luckily if you got lost there would be a Special Constable to guide you, no fear of being molested in those days, anyway not many males about as most were called up and occupied.

After six months I went on the District which I really enjoyed, I lived with the District Midwife, Mrs. Rayner, a widow, a lovely person nice and plump. Her two children were evacuated but she had a step-daughter Isabelle, 17 years of age who kept us both in order. We lived not far from the hospital and either walked to our patients or caught a bus, so plenty of exercise.

With our rations, which were very meagre, Isabelle gave us a good meal daily, at least I didn't have to eat conger eels, have never eaten one since after Thorpe Coombe food. We worked very hard and I had my first delivery on the District in a baker's shop, the flat above. Low beds were fashionable then, never should have been introduced, let alone divans. It was a double bed and had to kneel down to do the job. When I wrote home I said I never realized that jerries (chamber pots), brown paper and newspaper were so useful.

We occasionally relieved the few nurses round about in other areas, not often as not enough of us to cover the area where we worked. I loved the Cockney folk, even with great poverty and absence of appliances to use we never had ill treatment amongst the ordinary families. I dare say with all the toing and froing we delivered a lot of babies at home and seemed to visit for a longer time as no established Health Visiting at that time.

I suppose when I look back we had a hard time, but when 'let out' to practise our skills, we knew how to cope with any dire emergency when you could not get medical aid and as we say 'aint nature wonderful'.

We had an Andersons Air Raid Shelter in the back garden, which Belle had furnished with important kettle and paraffin lamp and heater so we had a cup of tea and biscuits. We did not use it very often at night as usually out, but anyway by the time we pulled and pushed Nurse Rayner in (the opening was very small and Belle and I were thin) and got settled down after great hilarity the all clear went and it started all over again.

I cannot tell you all that happened but sadly after my time on the District I was back on the Unit, then State Examination at Queen Charlottes. Written the first visit and then oral and practical. I don't think there were many failures and am sure due to the hostilities there had to be few more pushed through to carry on! Anyway having been asked to stay on at the Unit I decided I would come back to Norfolk, hopefully to go on the District.

After being at home for a break, the Inspector of Midwives, a Miss Davey from Norwich, rang my Aunt at the Nursing Home and requested me to go out on the District to relieve a nurse who had been taken ill. I arrived at Tilney and stayed at the *Shoreboat* Inn, a Public House, and took over until help arrived. They were lovely people at the *Shoreboat* and as I did not drive was handed a bicycle in rather poor condition. The nurse had a car, petrol was rationed of course. However, as it was evening time and a few bods were having their usual beers, they kindly pumped up the two leaking tyres and fixed up a pump so they could be kept up on my journey as there was a call out for me. I cannot remember where I went, but after one or two stops on the way, an event which I will not put in to print, made it. I did what I had to do and got back to the *Shoreboat* early hours of the morning. The landlord was more concerned about me not being fed so gave me the best meal I had had for a long time, country produce. I was eventually relieved by one of the Inspector of Midwives until a permanent one was found, so home again.

After another 48 hours I was requested or rather ordered to go to Wiggenhall St. Germans so the nurse could have her long overdue holiday. I stayed with a lovely family whom I knew, the Easters, had two weeks of good feeding, a good bicycle this time. In those days still no maternity unit, babies born at home but we had the General Nursing, Antenatal of Mothers, delivery and after care and Health Visiting as such. I didn't have many deliveries as many miscarriages due to the war activities and had a B.B.A. (born before arrival), not booked and Mr. Easter took me as he was home for his dinner, he was an Auctioneer. We had Yorkshire Pudding nearly every day, which I love. But nature was kind and the patient was safe and I just did what was necessary. It was strawberry time and we had a fete at their house and all in all was sorry to leave there.

After a couple of weeks went to Castle Rising to relieve the nurse for her overdue holiday. She and her sister lived in the nurses house which had been the Rectory in the past. I think I enjoyed my two weeks and had mostly general nursing to do, but had a very restful time really, just as well as did not know what was coming upon me next.

I was then sent to Docking, the nurse was taken ill. In fact she was nearly due for retirement and did not come back. I arrived out there, at least fetched as I had no car, one evening. I went to pick up the nursing bags from the Lady in charge of Nursing Association. She being very young and just had her second baby had a few little problems, like so many with babies. The bags were in a bad state with little or nothing in them, so wasn't very happy, especially as newly trained and being myself made a bad impression. However, I stayed at the *Hare Arms* Inn. Mrs. Jacobs was a nurse, although not officially practising, but had the same temperament as myself and was a great help getting my appliances together. The village chemist, Mr. Whitehead, was a great man and received me very well, because he just got moving to get what I needed, syringes, catheters, dressings and instruments which I hadn't got. He had a shop at Snettisham, I have never seen so many evacuees in these villages and we took over a largish house not in proper use to house the pregnant ladies and their families. The pubs did well.

We were situated near the Bircham Aerodrome, I didn't go there as the few married ladies who came with their husbands stayed at the *Hare Arms*, but went to their own homes when their husbands were posted. One couple newly married lived in Birmingham and we still keep in contact, unfortunately they did not have any children. The other couple from Southend had been married a couple of years, he like the others flew Hudson aircraft. Unfortunately Ted was posted south and she lived at home, by this time had had her first baby, a girl. He brought his plane back from a raid, made it to the coast but crashed. His crew were dead and he died very soon afterwards.

Miss Davey got a bit uptight when I demanded payment for my appliances. However, I said I would not stay unless I had the tools forthwith; that did it. She was against me living at the *Hare Arms*, not suitable for a nurse! Anyway as nobody came to take over was stuck there and went to live with Grace Playford in her little house near the *Hare Arms*, her husband was in the Army.

Well, what a life I led. A lot of premature babies which seemed to survive without all the carry-on we have now. It was the survival of the fittest in those days. I believe in it. I seemed to be out all the hours God sent, but I was very young. I had meals in various stopping places when I was a distance from home and tried to make the twice daily visits accordingly. We had a real snowed up winter and of course Docking and the area thereof got cut off with drifts very quickly, only one snow plough which would start out from Wells.

One night I had a lady in labour at Stanhoe and timed her for 4 a.m. approx. the next morning, so had to deal with Docking and get myself out there by 10 p.m. It was too dangerous to walk and of course could not ski, so called at an old farmer's house to see if I could borrow his cart horse, I won't go in to details, he was more concerned about his horse and not me. Having been brought up in the country I knew a horse would pave the way and not refuse to go, however, I arrived safely at midnight and the baby was born at about 3.30 a.m. A bit tricky, but after having two grown-up boys the mother was delighted with a lovely little girl.

WARTIME NURSING

During the scare of invasion, especially in that area, there were stone pill-boxes erected and controlled by the Home Guard. We had a good covering there and the head one was a Major from the 1914 War, he had an impediment in his speech and as I came home early one morning was suddenly confronted by him with fixed bayonet (the nearest I have been to one) and as I understood him he said 'Halt, who goes there'. I think he was not really awake because when I called him a silly old fool he discovered who he was prepared to stab. Bless him he looked so upset. Well, after a time I went to live at Bayfields butchers in the main road as their evacuees had taken off. Uncle Louis, he was a great character, his nephew became my husband in later years, used to live at Stoke Ferry, but used to cycle over to see me, needed his brains testing. I had no time for courting so sometimes never saw him. No petrol to come by van so he cycled back again. I was at Docking until a nurse arrived, after about 14 months I think. I came home with boxes of presents, china, etc., some of which I have still got, and was sorry to leave. Unfortunately by this time Miss Davey had got me all set to go out to Stow Vicarage, which the London County Council took over for evacuees and servicemen's wives to have their babies. It was the only place that had central heating, furnace I might say. The Vicar and his wife had retired and she was a wealthy American, hence the heating, although, apparently she kept extra warm with her 'tipple'.

I arrived out there in trepidation and was met by Miss Burrell who opened the premises, Aunty May greeted me with 'I hope you are used to hard work as you and myself are the only Midwives resident here. Three flights of stairs, my friend.' She is still my buddy, she was also the cook. We slept on the very top floor in the two attics, plenty of room but not much warmth, although there were fireplaces. The linen cupboard was between us and I have never seen such good equipment, plenty of everything and spares for influx patients which happened when people were bombed out, and it was good. The sheets and blankets went to Barretts Laundry each week, but all the rest was done on the premises.

This included napkins, baby gowns, patients' nightdresses and dressing-gowns, the dressing-gowns were American Red Cross towelling and good. I think by this procedure we never got infection, because the nighties and napkins had been in the copper. The bedpans were boiled once a day and of course our mothers were not allowed to go to the toilet until the 3rd day or longer. Just out of bed for bedmaking, but their toilet was done by the nursing staff. We had two wards, which had been the drawing-room and the dining-room near the front hall, the Labour Ward further down had been the breakfast-room and looked out onto the garden, very well equipped but only one labour ward bed. So we often delivered on the ward.

Aunty's May's desk was the other end of the hall, the medicine cupboard under lock and key half way and near a side entrance to the garden. Further along on the right was a lovely conservatory where we had our meals and through there a small room with toilet and basin for the patients who lived in the Day Room during the day, which used to be the Study and we and the mothers used to bath the babies in there as had a room attached. This was used in later days as the Village Hall, ideal for us as a long room and plenty of space for the babies as the nursery.

At the end of the house through a door was the kitchen area, the butler's pantry, or whatever it was, was used for the Baby Milk kitchen, where all the feeds were mixed as needed. The kitchen was very large with a large range for cooking and up two steps on the right two larders for storage of food, but at the back was the scullery where the vegetables were done. At the side was a bathroom and toilet, the maids' bathroom, only two maids, but we had to do the hand washing of blankets in there. We had linen lines outside but otherwise were dried on a pulley in the kitchen and scullery.

We had sometimes a Midwife on night duty, we took it in turns to help out as we had to do breakfast in the mornings, but much of the time Aunty May and myself had to do night duty when without a Midwife, the one and only had to leave as she could not go the pace!

We eventually had a Civil Nursing Reserve, like our Auxiliaries who had a few weeks training to help us, but she very often did night duty with us on call. All the patients who were delivered downstairs had to be carried up on a canvas stretcher afterwards. Then two downstairs wards were for waiting mothers, usually depending on how many. We had a steel shelter put in the drawing-room for getting the inhabitants in, as situated next to Bexwell Aerodrome and further from Marham.

During the day we had the Red Cross to help us, they were people in the nearby villages and we had one at a time. Although a Miss Peacock from South Runcton, one of three sisters, eventually came in daily and her sister who ran the estate came in on Saturdays and Sundays for about half a day. Wonderful they were, the other one came once or twice a week for a time – a Mrs. Haylett, she was great. They used to bring us titbits for the inner man to help out our rations. Although our Gladys, who was the cook and married to an airman was wonderful, she fed us with things nourishing out of very little. The old gardener did not approve of us lot being in his domain and hated making up the outside furnace to keep the heating going. We did it last thing at night. He hated parting with fruit and vegetables out of the garden, but we were also supplied from Stow Hall, which opened as a convalescent place for the wounded servicemen. There was no central heating there then, but it had big fireplaces and after the war when the Vicarage was given back to the clergy, the hall was opened for Midwifery by the Norfolk County Council as the new Unit, the first one, was being built at King's Lynn.

I spent three years at Stow and had a very happy time even with hard work and nights without sleep. The local Doctors came in to do the abnormal, except the Caesarean sections which went to King's Lynn, but happened very rarely as our patients were billeted in various villages and conveyed in by the W.V.S. and were vetted by a Mr. Bulman of Norwich who only died a few years ago, he was the Obstetrician and a wonderful man. We were lucky as he never made mistakes, you couldn't afford to do so in latter days and on the case notes of the people we dealt with was written warnings of any small snags that occurred. I wonder how long it will be before every person, especially mothers, are treated as individuals. As Mr. Arnold Walker in our training days said, 'Every pregnancy, labour and after care should be treated with great observation in all procedures and be ready for whatever presents itself to us unsuspecting mortals!'

When the heavy bombing started of course we had to take quite a number and up our bed occupancy to cope. We had Cockney folk, Servicemen's wives, all sorts of conditions but all seemed to get on together.

As usual a lot of ladies were confused over their date of expectation, but when we were getting over-full and knew those were near to date, we induced them with a dose of Castor Oil taken in lemon and it never did damage but worked if they were ready to part with their burden of trouble.

If we had premature or sickly babies who needed extra care, warmth and feeding, the large kitchen range gave plenty of warmth and all went well with them. Such a lot happened which I cannot tell you, but one incident was with a Welsh girl, married to a Cockney, she and her other child were billeted at East Dereham. She had a lovely singing voice and used to go round the villages singing and although she never talked to us very much, being a lady of few words, would render a song now and again. Well, she came in a bit earlier on with some raised blood pressure and hadn't a clue when she was due. In desperation one busy evening and being somewhat over-full we did the usual Antenatalling and for about the hundredth time asked her if she had any idea when she 'fell' for the baby, as it must be well ready. Before we could move a small voice said 'When the white bread change to brown!' Silence, and then Aunty May said to all the ladies 'count up'. When this happened amazingly, she was right and soon produced a mixed loaf! I reckon it was good for conception. If only we would listen to prospective mums a bit more, we wouldn't want a 'scanner'.

Ration books and ordering of food was done by Aunty May and our great cook Gladys Fox, who fed us with nourishing soups and puddings as there was very little meat. When Aunty May had to go away for a week and I had to do the catering I somehow ordered double rations! Oh my goodness, there was such a to-do. I was interviewed by various bodies (I couldn't have cared less) and in an ordinary situation could have been severely dealt with, but looking back and now older and wiser, realized there was no one to take my place, so no doubt that was the reason I was cautioned. We had to cut down on supplies on and off as the occasion arose to get back to normal.

We knew when the Invasion of Europe, Liberty D. Day, was for some time, as there was no news of the fathers of our babies (of course this happened during the five years of war, with only a few servicemen around to visit when on leave and not P.O.W.) So it was a bit hair-raising with the aerodrome activities going on more frequently, but we got through it. I had a quick marriage and was expecting a baby in 1945, I carried on until pretty latish and stayed for a few weeks with my Aunt and cousin in Sidney Street near the Maternity Home run by my Aunt Annie. My daughter Jennifer was delivered. I will not go in to details, but even being a Midwife I had a very bitter experience. When Jennifer was about two months old, she was born in the July, I went back to Stow, our cook was married to an airman who was sent to the East soon after their son's Christening. So the lad and Jennifer were brought up together at Stow for a space of time. Aunty May had to finish to go home to Beeston to care for her parents and eventually somebody came to take her place. I don't know how long she was there but she had not worked in our conditions.

I was hoping to set up house, my husband was a butcher with his brother and family at Stoke Ferry. As I had an operation to repair 'damages' my Aunt looked after Jennifer at the home, while I was in the Nursing Home concerned for surgery, etc.

I had hoped after recovery to go on the District, we still had very few Midwives. The Maternity Unit was being planned for the near future but Stow Hall was taken over for Maternity only, having had central heating installed.

I was asked to go on the District at Middleton, West Winch, West Bilney, Blackborough End and East Winch. Well spread out, the nurse had left rather suddenly; I don't blame her. I stayed with a very nice person, Mrs Rutterford, who ran the District affairs as the National Health Service had not started as such. She had two school age daughters and her husband worked in a bank in King's Lynn, I often wonder what happened to them after they moved away. My great friend who had been in the Land Army during the war (she died a short while ago) came to look after Jenny and then we moved to West Winch to live with an elderly lady. There was no nurses house, I think there was one, I was in charge really until someone came to take over. Eventually as time went by we went to live with somebody whom I knew, she and her husband had a small holding, fruit and vegetables. So there was room for us three at Blackborough End. It was very hectic and as usual I did not see much of my bed, I seemed fated to be a night bird and that is why I am in my 17th year of retirement. Still appreciate going to bed at night, when life is normal that is!

There was of course a lot of Midwifery still and of course as the servicemen came home an influx, we booked the mothers Antenatal and for the delivery, nursed them and did all the Health visiting and the General District Nursing. How we coped I do not know, but when you are young, I was now in my 30s and well broken-in, you just got on with it. I enjoyed it all, I was still cycling, petrol still rationed, but a nice gentleman taught me to drive in his spare time, the District car was a little Austin, I eventually had my own and you did not have to wait too long for a driving test, it had only just come into force. So after a short period of a few weeks my tutor said I could get going. I had a Provisional Licence of course, it must have been sheer luck and determination and a kind examiner that I passed, God help all. Folk who knew me kept their distance, I cannot tell you all that happened in the short time I was there. I had arrived as usual when there was heavy snow on the ground, a lot of problems and activities which I now put behind me. We were visited I think every three months by an Inspector of Midwives from Norwich. Isn't it marvellous when you need Midwives to deliver, etc., etc. the powers that be must have someone to go round with you to inspect!

I struck very unlucky just before I left, with one who expected you to be at your residence to take her with you on the round. We did not see eye to eye and on the last visit she came when I had been up all night, and still had two babies to bath. The air was thick with atmosphere I can tell you, I made her help me at each visit as she wished to leave by dinner time.

Just one item. I had a General Nursing Patient, a very nice body in her late forties with heart disease. Her eldest daughter, actually her niece who did her General Training with me, used to come over from Norwich when she could to help the seventeen-year-old daughter look after her mother. Nowadays she would have had heart surgery and done well, but even with treatment was full of fluid and in dire straits. We had a new doctor, Dr. Leakey, who was keen to get rid of the offending fluid, as there was no room at the hospital, and after getting a special Lawson Tate bed from London, that was a feat in itself. After the consultant told us what to do, he came out to see her after great preparations, dressing done for us at the chemists in King's Lynn, Mr. Bowskill, great man. Dr. Leakey did the small surgical operation and with luck and the good Lord keeping an eye on us, we drained off the fluid gradually.

In between other commitments, Dr. Leakey, myself and household managed to deal with various attacks. We dared her to die as a neighbour had spread round the village we were experimenting on her. However, mother Wright made great efforts and we had a good supply of liquid resuscitation and she recovered.

When we, myself and the Inspector of Midwives, arrived for what she thought was a first visit I had already been there in the early hours and prepared for the occasion and done her care. However, when the Inspector of Midwives saw the set up, after we had finished she took me aside and stated that it should never have been done at home and I was taking on far too many visits to my patients. So that did it and I am afraid I just let go, and didn't I feel better and said I would not be told when to visit my patients, etc., etc. and as there was someone to take over handed my resignation, written out that night. She disappeared in a hurry but not due to my words of rebuke, but something to do with a call of nature perhaps. I cannot divulge what had happened. However, our patient did recover and had a couple of years of quite happy living, so after all what does it matter. Actually I have always found that you get better results sticking to your guns. It is a pity they do not do so now, too many chiefs and not enough indians.

We were still directed as to where to practise, I think the powers that be thought we might all take off. So with my friend caring for Jennifer, left the District.

My friend took Jennifer to her home at Sedgeford for a break, while I was turning round. My Aunt now wanted to think about retiring, which she did. But the Obstetrician Mr. Harrison, a great character, asked her to go to the new Maternity Unit which had just been opened, and care for the babies. I in the meantime had been asked by the Brendan Stewart Nursing Home to finish off the Midwifery as they were taking Medical Patients as well. So as usual never said no.

This has been my downfall all my life. My friend Kathleen joined me and looked after Jennifer, now four years old and also helped to tend the sick patients, etc., I had a happy time there. Jenny was picked up on a Monday morning and attended a small private school run by the daughter of a farmer at North Runcton and became a weekly boarder. It was a good start for her as she gained her independence for future education, which I could see she would need to carry on at Boarding School later when she was 8½–9 years of age.

My sister-in-law, who used to keep house at the Stoke Ferry Butchery and looked after my husband, had previously, about four years ago, had a very large operation at Addenbrookes Hospital at Cambridge. Did very well really as she worked hard in the old big house. I would have liked to go back to District Nursing but miraculously that area had a Midwife, still of course doing General as well.

My Aunt retired from her Maternity Home and as the new Maternity Unit was then opening with little or no staff (as usual) I enjoyed a short time there. Unfortunately she had a fall and had some heart trouble so had to give up.

Going back into hospital was abhorrent to me now I had a 'leg free' and Stow Hall was running well for normal Midwifery, again with skeleton staff. It was the year of the Bulge with the males retiring from war Service to take on a 'new service' and the babies came I can tell you, still no clinics for birth control as such. So I was persuaded to go to the new Unit with a view to working at Stow Hall eventually. I was somewhat apprehensive I can tell you. It was a twenty-three bedded unit and mostly used for abnormal Midwifery. It was very well built considering the clamp down on building materials during the war, but if we had had more staff it would have been much easier. I have two great friends, retired Midwives living near me, and we have some very choice stories to discuss when we meet up now and then. One of them has been ailing for a long time and she was one of the first Sisters-in-Charge when the Unit opened, and although she has really been through the mill still comes up again and just as well as a very level headed person who will keep me under control with advice on how I should live! My other friend who is little in stature but with a big heart is my buddy and I hope so for a long time yet.

Well what a life we had! Our own theatre was not so big as the larger General Hospital to which we were attached. We had a flying squad, our consultant was now qualified as the Obstetrician Gynaecologist. A great fellow who worked day and night, even with a trained doctor and eventually a registrar. He went out on the District with one of us complete with equipment, plasma, sometimes blood, etc., broke the speed limit in his car, having had plenty of practice and you just sat tight. All sorts and conditions of course still in the homes, but we did what was necessary and the ambulance would carry the said victim S.O.S. but he would never let the patient travel in after haemorrhage, as in the past they died from shock and heart failure.

It worked well, being a man qualified to cope with any situation and a sense of humour. The Midwives, when available, would fetch the premature babies in S.O.S. and we eventually had a small portable Incubator with our equipment, which made life easier and went in an ambulance. It worked, and of course, I could write a book on funny experiences.

Our clinics were held in Outpatients, which we shared with the Gynaecology patients and their relatives. Usually Mr. Harrison did the Obstetric clinics Monday and Thursday mornings with his Gynaecology Consultant. The local Doctors sent them for vetting. The normal clinic was on a Thursday afternoon. We booked the mothers in in the early stages on a Wednesday, we had a wonderful secretary, Lily Large, she did the writing while we took the histories, anything abnormal was referred to Mr. Harrison Clinic, J.O.H. as he was known. It was a very good arrangement and no one was ever overlooked. It would be a great way of doing it these days and saved wasted money, our patients were sorted out right at the beginning and cared for by their own Doctors as was necessary, a lot of mothers still delivered safely at home, the population in full swing.

The Matron who ran the hospital was ex-army as the other lady retired. Having had no experience practising Midwifery, it sometimes made life very hard for us.

We, the few Midwives, flitted between the Unit and Stow Hall. I loved Stow Hall, although a mere handful of us with 30–32 bedded Unit and the usual flight of stairs, no lift, but it was a homely atmosphere. Two good Labour Wards with a sluice between and a nice Sterilizing Room, the dressings were done in a cellar, where there was an autoclave, this end of the hall was downstairs near the kitchen and other facilities, well thought out and equipped, although a lot of space to cover. The outside gardens and lawns were lovely for activities in the summer.

My first visit, I was sent in a hurry one evening as the elderly Sister was leaving; she actually did her General Training with me years ago, a bit older than myself, so expect she has gone on to higher things by now, wherever that is. It was absolute bedlam, myself on call to help the night Midwives with one helper Orderly. It was what you might call a 'hossing' night (Norfolk expression) and between delivering babies in quick succession, went into the kitchen to get a meal, keeping hot in the large Aga stove.

I heard a lot of squealing outside the kitchen window, which was open wide, it being hellishly hot, and when I looked out I saw a carpet of rats, large as life! I shut the back door and window and in the morning when I reported it to the Day Sister, she knew all about it. I will not go further, but when I reported it to the Matron, before hopefully I was going to rest, it was treated with no interest, so I informed her that we were liable to prosecution from the Health Authorities. However, it was sorted out and eventually the Pest

Control bloke arrived, but after a short time they were all back again. So Matron brought Blackie, the coal-black cat, who lived in the Nurses' Home at the General Hospital to keep the mice down. He had a rather secluded life and not very friendly, she let him out of the hamper and without warning he took a flying leap onto the big stove that cooked the puddings, and up to a big hole in the ceiling, which was the master entry to all the chimneys! What he did up there I don't know, but after 48 hours reappeared none the worse for his trip, he must have fed on something up there, then he took a long drink of milk and leapt out of the kitchen window.

After a short time he appeared with dead rodents laid out for us to see. That wasn't the only thing he caught, but he became quite friendly. The Gamekeeper was alarmed as to what would happen to the pheasant chicks he hatched out, but I don't think he ever caught one. He stayed with us a long time and kept the vermin away. Unfortunately he got caught in a trap (we think so) but he did have a good run. We missed him and the vermin came back again.

The Sister-in-Charge had gone, and as usual I carried on with great tribulation and skeleton staff and influx of babies, etc. and little or no sleep. We had no housekeeper, but a good cook and a few cleaners, then our cook became ill and after a pause, a chef came for a short time from our Isolation Hospital for a couple of weeks. In the meantime the post of Cook/Housekeeper was advertised; she arrived about six weeks before Christmas. I think she came from London, a little, quite elderly body who it turned out was quite fond of her tipple. However, she fed us well and were glad we didn't have to get on with housekeeping.

About 10 days before Yuletide it all happened. She got the stuff for making the Christmas Puddings and then one evening took off to King's Lynn in our transport van, which brought our requirements and arrived back about 9 p.m. When we and our cleaning ladies, who came in to practise Carol singing ready for our tour round the patients on Christmas Eve, she was very much incapable of walking (the taxi man brought her in) and we broke up the choir, carried her upstairs and put her in the Tower Room, a nice little room shut off and used in case of disaster. It has been said it was haunted, I didn't know, but when I hoisted our Union Jack on the balcony very firmly I might add, in commemoration of some Royal occasion, the damn thing would not stay up and it never did, but that is just by the way. We locked her in with facilities for toilet use and I telephoned the Matron, who of course, did not believe me and said get her doctor, luckily it was the good bloke who helped me on the District and we got a urine specimen which smelt of good old rum, so he knew whether to sedate her or not, we didn't of course, by this time she was snoring. I went to bed at 3 a.m. and instructed the Midwife on night duty not to let her out, and if any trouble call me.

Well about 5 a.m. she was hammering on the door and kicked up a hell of a din, the two staff were petrified and patients upstairs. So I got dressed after a sleepless night, unlocked the door and was greeted with much abuse for locking her up in a haunted room. I escorted her to do her ablutions and left her in care of the Orderly as I was needed in the labour wards.

I telephoned the Matron who said she would be out to see her and I suggested she made it mighty quickly in case she took off! Which of course she did and the last we saw of her was trotting down the drive, one of the day cleaning ladies saw her thumb a lift, I don't know where.

She left a note saying she would like her belongings sent on and her salary, I can't remember the address. I will not go into details about my conversation with Matron, but told her maybe I could find someone to take over.

My friend Kath was finishing at Brendan Stuart Nursing Home and Jennifer at Boarding School, so I rang her up and said I would tell the Matron she would come in a week's time as we were desperate. She came and in the meantime, the staff between us coped with the food; good job the kitchen was near the Labour Ward!

With Christmas on the doorstep we had to make the puddings, so the cleaning ladies and a Staff Midwife, who helped us on Sundays came in. We found the ingredients and had a hilarious time with a bit of help from the mums, we all had a stir and a wish, it smelled well of beer, etc., and in they went in the big steamer to cook. I went to bed around midnight, and requested the useless Midwife on night duty just fill up the steamer S.O.S. She called me early a.m. and I smelled the puddings! So before flying into the Labour Ward had a look, no water, boiling dry. However, I added water and hoped for the best, then did my duties in the Labour Ward, etc., but kept an eye on the puddings! They were all right on the day, so felt we had done a great job.

My friend Kath arrived and plunged right into it, she was housekeeper, etc. for a good few years until the Hall closed. She has joined all the folk up to higher things just recently.

Well a very nice, fairly elderly Sister came and took over full charge, we worked together for a time, I hoped for a long time, she was delightful, getting nearer to retiring age. We had a Garden Fete while we were there, a lovely day and plenty of help. I missed the opening, much to Matron's disgust, but my friend Sister Allen and I delivered a baby which was loath to come, but the mother well remembers how we chivvied her on so she could see a bit of the fete from the ward window!!

Well, our Sister left, we were very sad, but she had so much criticism from higher authority, unwarranted, so will say no more.

Luckily we had 1½ Midwives on night duty for a time as I got fed up and was hoping for someone to come and take charge, as I was overdue to go back to the Unit.

One memorable day and night we had so many admissions and deliveries, we ran out of cots and laundry, so after getting up at 4 a.m. to help the Midwives, rang the Matron and asked for equipment as so desperate, I didn't get a proper answer, she did say she would do what she could. So in the end I rang the Unit and eventually J.O.H. and my friend B. Baker, Sister-in-Charge, came out with what they could carry and the ambulance followed with beds!

We managed to get the labouring mums into accommodation, they stayed to help us with the suturing, etc. until we saw daylight. There was a funny side to it, and we took it all in our stride. Ah me, what days, we were younger then, then off I went, back to the Unit. Part of it was closed for renovation and repairs, so another bout of chaos, which I prefer to forget. On top of that the Sister-in-Charge, my friend B., was leaving. Having had a belly full of all the hassle she went to London to do administration and eventually became Matron at Market Harborough Hospital.

This left us with one Midwife on night duty, one full-time and one part-time on day duty.

I was never asked to run the unit and didn't want to, as I wanted to be free of hospital. The day B departed I still did not know I would be left. By this time the Matron was trying to close Stow Hall for Midwifery, eventually after repairs were done and with a view for extension of the premises, I was told I could carry on. Being occupied in our theatre, unable to see the Matron to say no, but later in the day did so. She was advertising for a Sister-in-Charge, so I told her to move heaven and earth, so I will go no further. But as it is not the thing of course I did not walk out, but carried on until we got someone.

That is another chapter, so I will continue to just describe very briefly the six-year struggle with three full-time Midwives for Day and Night Duty, and one or two part-time staff who we were very dependent upon. By this time Stow Hall was closed, mysteriously, to Midwifery and kept for Convalescent patients; which was greatly appreciated by hundreds of people and used as the modern description (to its full potential), I hate that word, but it certainly covers a lot of devious excuses for little staff for the great job it did.

Myself, I feel that my potential was gained. Like us all then there was unpaid overtime, which we did not mind of course, but it was the usual loss of sleep. You may be amused but my great joy, even now after retirement, is getting to bed at a normal time, half an hour read and eating a daily apple. I do not like the taste of over-rated toothpaste at night (I still have my own teeth to eat with) and there has only been peace for the last 1½ years, even after 13 years of retirement, sadly lost nearly all my family, I do not feel lonely, there is no time.

Gradually equipment improved: 1, 2, 3, incubators for the premature and sick babies, our first small portable one cost then £100+ bought by voluntary money to fetch the District ones in.

Life was still very rough on the District, but eventually we had our unit, bed and ward numbers increased, not the Labour Ward end which was good equipment, we had to use one of the Labour Wards as a theatre S.O.S.: no problem, just a bit of furniture moving. We all enjoyed our job even with high-up interference. It is now lovely looking back, realizing how the daft short-sighted Government kept changing and introducing various high class named new reports. The only one and the first for us was the Cranbrooke Report sponsored by Lord Cranbrooke. We had our meeting periodically with District people represented, especially the Inspector of Midwives who visited the Unit to sign the usual books and it was a pleasure to see her, because our liaison with the District was a great asset. Still only a few Midwives in most areas.

The new Units training Midwives in other hospitals I think logged most of them, but life was getting saner, I think. I still seemed to be always fighting with higher authority, but this is how we kept going. You will never get anything done rightly, unless you fight for it, and I still think when you yourself know what is so, just stick to your guns. I did and still would do it and if I know I was in the position not to get 100% results, would sink down and never put our mothers and offspring at risk.

Our Consultant J.O.H., was wonderful, not always popular but nothing was ever changed without he went into each detail and always saw every patient's notes eventually; and kept the written records which we had to do to the minimum, but every detail was important and I can see now why dealing with emergencies. Still I could relate a lot of queer things which used to happen, but it kept us on our toes and even without machinery (which is used today). Our powers of observation were used to think full potential, I think you get a sixth sense somehow. Yes, we were often overtired, but I suppose we were encouraged by our mothers, I mean it.

THE NEW MATERNITY WING

Before entering onto the new life, spent in a new Maternity Unit being designed and built, I will describe what a great time we had at Christmas, never off duty of course. But a few weeks before we got our heads together to design and decorate our Unit. No streamers allowed because of fire risk, I don't like them anyway, but we used all sorts of stuff (I will not say where it all came from), but we had a wonderful Doctor's wife who had been a Midwife coming in a few evenings each week and she supplied us with all sorts of unlikely things. One year she managed to get us some fishermen's nets to trim the front lobby and piles of shells. We made a lighthouse for the front corridor and had all the assets which we painted from drawing paper and put on cardboard and cut out and trimmed the patients' bed lights with shades depicting the ocean, etc. Everybody, including the mothers, were kept busy doing things for us. We all had great fun in between delivering numerous babies. Christmas Eve I joined in with the General Staff with Carols, complete with lanterns. There was one Sister who ran the Ophthalmic Department, she had a lovely soprano voice and in the elated high pitched Carols, we rested our voices and let her carry the music. I am afraid she has sadly gone to higher things, I hope she keeps her voice in trim in case I join her (with luck when I have repented my sins) but I hope it will be a little longer so I can catch up with what I have left undone, i.e. visiting.

We were still depleted of staff, but always were on the way; myself now 46 years of age and getting a bit weary of high up problems. I made a remark one day that I had had it, even if I became pregnant, which of course I did in between joining my husband, who was still in business for occasional visits, life was still chaotic for many of us. Jennifer was 17 years old and studying with a view to go on to college (I think I put her off nursing and medicine, maybe). Plans had to be made for the future, advertisements went in again for a future Lady-in-Charge. I think the lady higher up was somewhat pleased with our problems, as she thought she would persuade my two stalwart colleagues to do it. But like myself they just wanted to care for the mothers and babies and did not fancy being controlled by untrained Authority. I realized all was not well with me, but we carried on and managed to get up to date before I was due to finish.

In the meantime we lost two Aunts within 10 days of each other. My cousin Emmie had a flat which she had taken for a year so as she was on her own. My husband being 10 years older than myself might retire. Helen arrived, a few weeks early, a friend of our family, a Methodist had bought a house but would only let it to us, and that was just after Helen arrived. As I had such problems with Jennifer it was decided I would be delivered Caesarean Section. I stayed with my cousin at her flat to be near at hand and get my dental appointments up to date and other things. I had ordered provisionally a complete layette for Helen from Joshua Taylor at Cambridge until I was sure of a baby. I still think that most mothers know when all is not normal within them, and if only the powers that be would listen to them a bit more life would be easier. They can still have reassurance. Well in the early hours of a Sunday morning in October 1962 it began, my cousin came with me the few yards we had to go to the Unit.

Still only one Midwife on night duty, God help us, so one of us had to get things at night. When I arrived my two friends looked at me, I will not go into the conversation. The theatre which had been cleaned up was got ready. Our Consultant, J.O.H. was away but expected home on the Monday, but we had a good Indian Registrar and two anaesthetists around. I suggested I felt, I will use the Norfolk expression, 'like Barney's Bull', but of course must invent one for the female species. However, by about 6 a.m. J.O.H. arrived. I don't know how far he had come from but saying my last words before being shut up, about him coming hot haste, he looked worse than I did, but right fast Helen arrived. I do not know what went on, and glad I didn't because things were a bit complicated. I can remember my two friends tidying me up and apparently the conversation was, let us wake her up to do the cleaning up. What a pity I could not answer.

I cannot remember much until my husband called in the afternoon and I saw him double and went to sleep again. But on Monday sometime when I was sat up, Helen was brought to me by one of the lovely nursing people. A mother herself, I just looked at Helen and knew she was as I thought, a Downs' Syndrome infant, but she was beautiful to look at. However, she had to be specially cared for and so spent her first six weeks up and down. But I went to Stow Hall for a couple of weeks convalescence, which prepared me for the future.

My cousin, with help, got the house ready and I sent for the layette for Helen. The carry cot was given to me by our staff. Really it was lovely to get all without the coupon problem that I had with Jennifer.

During this time, while I was getting my second breath, I had an invitation to a celebration of the Centenary of the Midwives Board in London, which of course is now the Royal College of Midwives. It is sad to think that this was altered as it was a body of people who controlled the complete running of the Midwifery Profession, with no political interference. Rules and Regulations and the asset of our own treasurer. Only a few great people, but respected by us and the Medical Profession. The affair was being held at the Royal College of Gynaecologists and Obstetricians, and attended by the Queen Mother, who has been our patron for a long time. I was not too happy about going, but I was persuaded by my colleagues to do it. So I was taken up to London by my friend (God rest her soul) and stayed by invitation of the Matron at the Royal Northern Hospital, where my friend who used to run our Unit was now on the Administrative staff at the hospital. We stayed in the Nurses' Home for the two nights. I was decked out in suitable dressage, most of it borrowed as I had lost a great deal of weight. I was seen off with a great ceremony in a taxi to be at the said gathering by 6.30 p.m. In a Norfolk accent the driver asked me where it was situated, of course being clueless. I had an idea it wasn't far from the zoo. He got on the blower, we had a goodish, hilarious journey, he came from King's Lynn, delivered me safely and said he would willingly pick me up at 10 p.m. to take me to the Palladium, my two colleagues had complimentary tickets, me going in at half-time.

We were received by Arnold Walker, my lecturer, now the Chairman of the C.M.B. and Professor Alan Moncrief, who I had had tuition from in times gone by. There were 200 'Madwives' from all over the country, and each county group, two from each county, were aptly looked after and plied with good fluid until the Queen Mother arrived at 7 p.m. I think that our medical males were having a wonderful time and kept us all well entertained, including the Consultant to the Royal Family at that time, 1962. The Queen Mother moved around and spoke to us all, all in all I had a very entertaining evening. We had a buffet meal and drinks and then I went to the Palladium for the second half of the show and met up with my friends. We went for an evening meal before retiring back to the Nurses Home, about 2.30 a.m. The next day, as my friend B had a day off, we went shopping and then travelled back to King's Lynn the next day.

After all the excitement my cousin and myself with helpful friends settled in the house where I live now. Went and brought Helen home on December 14th when the first snow came and we had the most dreadful frozen up winter I can remember. Poor Helen who had now decided to survive despite ups and downs was confined to the house until the end of April and early May, when the last icy conditions departed and we then had the hottest summer during my life time. My cousin Emmie, who I nicknamed the landlady, as she still bossed me around (having helped to rear me and did not think much of Nursing Profession bods) cared for Helen and with some domestic help I returned to the Unit on night duty. Still skeleton staff, one or two creeping in. Although still doing 12 hours on duty seven days with two nights off weekly, we struggled on. As I was now 47 years old I thought about retiring as soon as the staff situation improved.

The new Maternity Unit was being built, what a monstrosity, miles of corridors hither and thither, I took my bicycle on duty one night just to see if I could get from A to B a bit quicker. Unfortunately the corners were a problem, they all had to be reinforced eventually, not my fault, as I only did the round twice on a bike, as I couldn't see what was coming round the corner.

Well, now with a new Salmon Report operating, instead of a Sister-in-Charge a lady arrived called the Principal Nursing Officer, responsible for furnishing etc. of the new Unit.

We, the few staff, had to apply for our posts as Midwives. Now can you imagine how my colleagues and myself of quite advanced years felt. We received application forms and you will never believe this but they were the same forms with a few extra bits and pieces as when I, now in my fifties, had duly filled in years ago. Well, as my three colleagues were going 'up there' it **was** up I can tell you, I decided to try it all out. I filled in my form with great gusto, no references as most people had passed on. I will not go into it any further! I was prepared for the worst.

The night before the great 'exodus' was one I will never forget, I was sorry our Consultant J.O.H. had retired, it was sad but he was very practical, but we were lucky with our new one, Miss McGaskill, Scottish and wonderful with her lovely accent.

Luckily we had two Midwives on duty, my steady hard working humorous buddy (she has sadly passed on to higher things), and that night we had nine babies born and other emergencies and believe it or not we ran out of equipment! I will not go into any more details, but by the morning it was chaos. Mothers and babies taken up by ambulance in relays and the last one left, very near to delivering with expected complications, however, she travelled and the good Lord kept his eye on her, and more by luck than management she just made it.

I went home, fell into bed after a hot bath and went on duty to the new abode. I was in charge of the ward, the Delivery Suite, a new midwife, Labour Wards separate and infant S.C.B.U. run by my colleague, Emma, in between.

What a night finding everything. As we had microphones on our old unit, it was very feet saving. But the new unit had old fashioned buzzers and as there were 46 bedded wards and 12 single rooms it was like a marathon, waste of space and time and precious energy, equipment not where it should be, etc., etc. However, after helping in the Labour Ward on and off I survived the night, being still agile in my fifties and eventually 60. By the time I was 62 we were pretty well staffed, considering. Eventually due to other snags another report was introduced (I can't remember what it was called). As new equipment arrived gradually to improve conditions and aid for the mothers, the babies still came when not planned for.

The powers that be tried to get the babies in to the world in the daytime as much as possible; who thought that one up, I don't know. But nature wins in the end and now these days things are slowing down with experimentation to do otherwise, but the Midwife situation is not good, it grieves me.

In commemoration of our Queen's 25 years on the Throne, God help her, various people were sent a silver medal and scroll for service. Quite out of the blue, I came home one morning on my knees to be greeted with a torn envelope (it was at the time when letter bombs were fashionable). My cousin took it in, as I was busy with my chores before going to bed and visiting a dear old lady near us, giving her daughter help, my cousin shouted oh oh you have got a medal. I didn't stop and look and read, as I was rather busy, but as it turned out it was a medal. I replied waste of money, the money could have been used for a bed pan trolley which we hadn't got. News travels fast (not from myself), as I do not approve of medals. When I went on duty and took the report I was asked to show the medal, after a visit by our P.N.O. was requested to meet the *Lynn News & Advertiser*. To be photographed in the morning.

Having started to re-drive a car at 60 years of age I had acquired *Bessie*, my Vauxhall Viva. With the help of our porter I took off like a bat out of hell down the by pass as I had a hair appointment. So I managed to get out of that one, I felt rather sorry as I saw the lad parking his car as I slid out.

Well, life carried on as hectic as ever, Helen improved slowly and became a great joy to us and all our friends and neighbours. I will not dwell on the next few years, but we all felt we were running in the marathon!

I was still happy caring for the mothers and babies. We eventually got more staff, and a tutor as we became a Midwifery Training School, so had pupils, not many. What was so unnecessary was extra writing to do.

One new report which was introduced advocated much less pen

pushing, etc. by practising Midwives. J.O.H. Case Notes were scrapped but as he very wisely said: if there were simpler and 100% correct notes there would be no slip ups at all. Life and security for all of us staff and patients would be guaranteed. Well, I approached my 62nd birthday and began to slow up! I had done two extra years, the staff situation was well and truly established, I retired and looked forward to a bit of peace, plenty of sleep and for the first time in my life I was able to take up the running of a household.

RETIREMENT (NEARLY!)

My husband, who died after a short illness in 1971, never retired, although he was 65 years of age. The butcher's business was sold, his brother retired; he was older than my husband. My sister-in-law, who kept house, had died previously to this. My daughter No. 1, Jennifer, had been married a year, she and her husband are both school teachers. Helen, by this time in her ninth year, and attending the Alderman Jackson School for children with special needs. Lovely lady in charge and her staff, a very happy place. Jenny and spouse were here with me as they were on holiday from school, in August, when my husband died. They were able to take over the household as I was still working, it was a bad time, luckily my cousin and Helen were staying with my niece at Mundesley. Just as well as my cousin still treated me as an inexperienced individual, unable to cope with death and all the etc. which go with it, but we managed very well, I think. Just as well because after a great celebration send-off for my retirement, plenty of trouble ahead.

Before anything could happen my cousin and myself had a coach tour to Scotland, actually right up to a year before she died at 86, she and her friend had a holiday every year and sometimes twice and she was still boss of the house.

As soon as I got my feet on the ground along came a Male Health Visitor, Mr. Booth, to help with a few other folk, one who is two years older than myself, and still our secretary, and another lady, Mrs. Ward, also a Health Visitor to get together a group of handicapped adults who he had rounded up just sitting at home as there was no room for them at the Training Centre just opened. We had so many, but the Sorenson Car Factory put a car into a race I believe and gave us £650 to start us off. As we had no premises the Catholic

Father let us have the school room attached to his Church. It worked temporarily, but of course we needed more heated accommodation for our needs. So dear old Mr. Goldsworthy, who created the St. Raphael Club, and was the retired Relieving Officer, took us in. We were still a Voluntary Organization, but eventually after some time formed a committee and were financed partly by the State via Social Services and Council.

Mr. Booth was now satisfied with the Adult Centre, by now working in co-operation with the North Lynn Training Centre. Suddenly without warning he approached me with a view to setting up a Mothers and Toddlers mixed group, mainly for children in need of help, mind you having the mothers as well worked well I think, as they shared with each other and us their problems. We had permission from the Gayton Road Health Centre, no rent to pay, and other powers to have a room there, after 14 years we are still doing it. Actually it is still organized chaos. But the staff and the doctors at the centre are fabulous. Of course there was another report brought forth (it keeps the politicians quiet even if they are up the spout). Mr. Booth is due I suspect for higher things, but I fear he could have been a thorn in the flesh for the higher ups, but he and Mrs. Ward were wonderful, even if I haven't forgiven them for leaving me holding the baby. I didn't know much about handicapped children but have learned by experience mighty fast since!

I was requested by various people like the W.I., bless them, British Legion, Good Companions and the rest to talk to them and would be given a small donation to keep my lot going. I have enjoyed doing it although it is a bit time consumimg. But it enables me to meet many of the mothers, and now grandmothers, whom I 'bullied'.

I am sorry I do not go to the Wisbech gatherings, but do not like driving a distance at night. Even with carrying weapons for self-defence, I am more concerned I might lose my car, as I could never afford another one. You get attached to your vehicle.

Well, after various little problems with Helen's health and giving help to various members of my family and coping with the setting up of affairs, that is the bugbear, but I am getting used to it, I am still on the committee for our Adult Centre, although unable to go in and help. But I have been on quite a few of their holiday trips to various holiday camps, which are enjoyable hard work. My Toddler Group and the Mad Mothers as I call it, each summer holiday when the rest of the family break up school we have a large bus and enjoy our three or four trips to various parks, where there is entertainment for all and sundry, and we take everything but the kitchen sink with us. We also celebrate all our little ones birthdays, we are a small group, we had to be as it is a starting point for mothers with problems, before they go to school. I hope it will continue after I pass on and hopefully some unsuspecting soul will do it, established properly, hence all the pen pushing.

After a few family deaths, my cousin the landlady who was a great pillar of our Chapel and sang in the choir for years, and also played the organ until some few years ago until her arthritis got the better of her. She remained Secretary of the Afternoon Townswomen's Guild and lots more until she had to succumb to inactivity, except her brain and tongue. She took herself to bed and said she longed to die as she was no good to anybody, there was a funny side to it.

I remember her telling the Doctor when she agreed to see him, and he said, 'well you are in good hands which will help me'. She said 'that is what you think. If I had to listen to her (that is me) I should have been dead long ago!' When I saw the Doctor out I said 'now you have heard it all'. My great friend and colleague Emma helped to look after her for 10 weeks and the District people the last two weeks. My Helen missed her and was going somewhat downhill and seemed to gradually get worse after losing her favourite Nemmie, as she called her; she only required me, her mother when she was ill.

Then we had a heart-breaking month when she rapidly became unable to visit her friends and neighbours and then on Tuesday night she had violent pain and a perforated duodenal ulcer. I took her into hospital and stayed all night and part of the next day. I will not go into any more detail as it became a nightmare as there had to be a post-mortem after she died that day at about 1.30 p.m. I had no time to grieve as I had all the telephoning to do, but I was well supported by neighbours and friends as there were no relatives near. She had a great send off, Chapel full of people and the choir and it was a very happy occasion for us all to thank the Almighty for all the joy she brought to so many of us. I feel I have lost my family now, her ashes are in Nemmie's grave at the little village cemetery at Wereham where I was brought up, and one day I will be with them both. I am only upset when I see the Children in Need and all what happens abroad, and I only regret that I am not younger to go out and do a bit to love and care for them.

I just hope that the younger generation will be able to read this book and realize that my generation are responsible for what is happening today. Also this is a lovely world and should not be abused by greed and lust or money. The young generation are growing up and aiding in their own way to make a better land for us. We are proud of our Country, and people who want to live in harmony, work hard, never kill anybody I might add, let us tell them it is the right thing to marry and have families, but give them discipline, which you hardly need if they have care and love from their parents. A baby is a person and aware of the mothers' feelings as soon as they are born. Each one is an individual and needs help and advice, even after they leave the nest. They are the priority and if the parents do not want a child, well they do not need to these days do they?

Do you know I never realized until these last years that when a child looks at you, they know what goes on in your mind and if they can trust you. I wonder if we ever get a second chance to make up for all the mistakes we have made in this life.

I believe there must be a hereafter or whatever you may call it, because although our loved ones have gone, there is something around which if you are doing something you shouldn't and that is still often with myself, even now in my latter days and I still feel guilty, cross myself and do the right thing.

I do think and hope that when my time has come that I can sit in the chair, shut my eyes and go to sleep, no hassle with complaints which need a lot of you know what, maybe I can say in Norfolk dialect. This is it, to hell with all the hassle you lot 'git on with it' I am 'orf' and hope to catch up on me sleep. I wonder?

Tell me not in mournful numbers,
Nursing is a lovely dream.
I'm half sick from lack of slumbers,
Things are never what they seem.
Doctors, Nurses, Sisters, Patients,
Thou' my heart be stout and brave.
Yet their trying ways will send me
Very shortly to my grave.
Getting into lots of trouble,
Rows and ructions day by day.
Getting blamed for faults of others,
Tons of work and little pay.
Yet at the end of all these troubles
What at last will be my fate.
Like a broken down old Cart Horse
Rest will come, but Ah! too late.

HOW TRUE